Shark Cartilage

by Rita Elkins

Woodland Publishing
Pleasant Grove, UT

The information in this book is for educational purposes only and is not recommended as a means of diagnosing or treating an illness. All matters concerning physical and mental health should be supervised by a health practitioner knowledgeable in treating that particular illness. Neither the publisher nor author directly or indirectly dispense medical advice, nor do they prescribe any remedies or assume any responsibility for those who choose to treat themselves.

© 1996 Woodland Publishing

Woodland Publishing
P.O. Box 160
Pleasant Grove, UT
84062

CONTENTS

THE SHARK: A SPECIMEN OF
REMARKABLE HEALTH . . . 5

THE CASE FOR SHARK CARTILAGE AS A
CANCER THERAPY 13

CASE STUDIES USING SHARK CARTILAGE
FOR ARTHRITIS 20

MEDICINAL APPLICATIONS OF
SHARK CARTILAGE 28

ENDNOTES 31

THE SHARK: A SPECIMEN OF REMARKABLE HEALTH

Sharks have been called the earth's only perfect living creatures. Strong, agile, disease resistant and incredibly fast, they have created both fear and admiration in the human mind. While none of us would like to venture too close to these magnificent predators, they may hold the key to controlling some of the most devastating diseases we currently face as a society.

Unquestionably, sharks are specimens of magnificent health. They possess a potent immune system which, unlike ours, is supported by the consistent presence of circulating antibodies. These defensive entities are ready to attack at the very moment an unwanted invader threatens infection. This highly efficient immune system promotes rapid wound healing and provides superior infection protection.

As a result of their extraordinary physical prowess, sharks live an extremely active life, unhampered by the types of disease that afflict man. Why? What differentiates the two organisms? What bio-enhancing secrets does shark physiology hold? Modern scientists have only begun to discover that this 400 year old creature may pose its most significant threat to an unexpected prey: cancerous tumors. Surprisingly, it is the seemingly benign cartilage frame of the shark that holds its most impressive medicinal promise

Secrets of Shark Cartilage

The shark is an unusual sea creature whose endoskeleton is made entirely out of cartilage rather than bone; a fact that differentiates sharks from other land or sea creatures. Cartilage is a tough material composed of protein and carbohydrates, and unlike bone, contains no blood vessels or nerves. In the human body, cartilage acts as a protectant "pad" between moving bones, comprises the Adam's apple, top of the ear, supports nasal tissue, and constitutes various "tubes and pipes" found throughout the body. Cartilage has the remarkable ability to provide support and protection without the benefit of nourishment from blood vessels or nerves. It receives life-giving nutrients via body fluid or water, which is enhanced by body movement. For this reason, a lack of physical activity can deprive cartilage of water, thereby initiating a process called calcification, which turns flexible cartilage into a hard, stony material.

Shark cartilage is unusually abundant and contains specific compounds which set it apart. It contains ample amounts of certain biological substances which keep it vessel free. These are the bio-chemicals which give shark cartilage its impressive therapeutic value. Simply stated, shark cartilage is capable of inhibiting tumor growth and reducing pain.

The Chemical Composition of Dried Shark Cartilage

Chemically speaking, shark cartilage is a combination of proteins and complex carbohydrates called mucopolysaccharides. A quick perusal of its chemical constituents does not reveal the presence of any magical compounds, however, it chemical structures and synergistic actions provide significant therapeutic actions. The arrangement of its protein molecules creates a potent effect which has profound implications for a whole host of devastating diseases.

ash	41 percent
(60 percent calcium and phosphorus)	
protein	39 percent
carbohydrate	12 percent
water	7 percent
fiber	<1 percent
fat	<0.3 percent[1]

The Struggle to Find a Cancer Cure: A Losing Battle?

While medical science has made tremendous strides in new and impressive ways of putting broken bodies and torn flesh back together, its approach to the treatment of certain diseases has been inefficient to say the least. Conventional therapies prescribed for cancer and arthritis can be toxic, tortuous, and in many cases, ineffective. In choosing the best method of disease treatment, it was Hippocrates who admonished, "First, do no harm." Most of these therapies weaken and cripple the immune system in attempting to eradicate disease. In addition, the use of harmful chemotherapy and radiation take a tremendous toll on healthy tissue. Moreover, potent pharmaceutical drugs are frequently used too mask symptoms and rarely address the origin of the disease.

The purpose of this booklet is not to discourage anyone suffering from cancer or other diseases like arthritis to evaluate or use standard medical treatments. It does, however, wish to discuss the viability of a specific alternative therapy called shark cartilage, which works with, rather than against the immune system. Shark cartilage does not fall into the category of faddish or unsubstantiated alternative therapies. The potential of shark cartilage for treating devastating degenerative diseases has been and continues to be well-documented. Its potential for treating cancerous tumors, however, remains relatively untapped.

In 1990 alone, over one million people were diagnosed with cancer. Worse yet, predictions for the future are nothing less than appalling. It is estimated that eventually, one out of every two of us will develop some form of cancer. Despite millions spent on the quest for a cure, cancer continues to claim an inordinate amount of life. Treating cancer has usually focused on destroying tumors through invasive procedures which in and of themselves can be life-threatening.

Unfortunately, promising non-toxic therapies like shark cartilage for cancer are usually passed over as nothing but quackery by the cancer researchers who are quick to dismiss them as unproven and meritless. Scientists are slow to acknowledge the value of substances they don't recognize as their own: an attitude which has left them red-faced on more than one occasion. For decades, health advocates have preached the vital importance of a low fat, low animal protein, high fiber, high fruit and vegetable diet as the best mix for longevity and disease prevention. Likewise, the use of vitamin C, vitamin E, B-complex, acidophilus, selenium and a whole host of other supplemental nutrients have been discussed by naturopaths for their remarkable curative properties.

Today, medical practitioners are vigorously touting the benefits of diet and the use of supplements like folic acid to promote health. Even controversial treatments for cancer like visualization therapies are employed by a growing number of medical practitioners who are finally acknowledging a profound link between the mind and the body. The admission that diet and vitamins play a profound role in determining health, however, has been slow in coming. Unfortunately, precious time has been wasted. By the time medical science admits that an alternative treatment shows solid clinical activity, hundreds of lives have been lost to unsuccessful but accepted methods of treatment.

Shark cartilage has already emerged as a non-toxic treatment for cancer and other diseases. For the last several decades, its ability to inhibit the growth of tumors and stimulate the immune system have been scientifically documented. Read for yourself. Nature has provided shark cartilage with powerful but non-toxic medicinal compounds, capable of treating not only cancer, but arthritis, psoriasis, and other degenerative diseases as well. In addition, shark cartilage can act as an effective preventative against the development of these diseases.

NOTE: This booklet in no way advocates abandoning orthodox medical treatments for diseases like cancer. It provides information on the value of shark cartilage in order to inform the consumer of its possible potential. Shark Cartilage can and should be used in conjunction with other standard therapies.

Do Sharks Get Cancer?

For decades, scientists have wondered why sharks have such a low rate of cancer development. In his book, *Sharks Don't Get Cancer,* Dr. I. William Lane discusses the relatively rarity of shark carcinomas. He believes, and with good cause that, "one reason why sharks are so long-lived is they are one of the few living creatures that almost never get cancer. It now appears that the abundance of cartilage in sharks may explain why these fish are not prone to cancer..."[2] It is the presence of certain biochemicals found in shark cartilage which inhibits the growth of tumors even when sharks are exposed to massive amounts of extremely carcinogenic substances.[3]

Dr. Lane has stated:

> ... some cancer has been reported in sharks, but fewer than one in a million sharks show cancer ... less than 1 percent of the incidence of tumors reported for all other species of fish. What is relevant is that sharks rarely get cancer and that this fact has been tied specifically to their cartilage skeleton

and the strong anti-tumor activity of shark cartilage . . . Six to eight percent of a shark's weight is cartilage, which is about 1,000 times the amount of cartilage found in a calf of the same weight. Also, shark cartilage is slightly different from that of other mammals.[4]

The following quote refers to the impressive ability of sharks to fight off infection and carcinogens:

The shark's immune system has a large amount of antibodies always circulating; so, there is no 'lag time' before going into battle. These antibodies are so powerful that sharks almost never develop common infections (even in the most unsanitary conditions). In fact, their chances of developing cancer are less than one in a million.[5]

A ten year survey of sharks at the Mote Marine laboratory in Sarasota, Florida revealed that sharks exposed to high doses of carcinogens never developed tumors of any kind.[6]

For over 400 million years, these creatures have remained relatively free from a disease that has killed scores of human beings.

Shark Cartilage: The Best Natural Treatment for Cancer?

Shark cartilage has the remarkable ability to destroy tumors by preventing the creation of blood vessels which nurture and sustain tumor growth. Richard Passwater, Ph.D. refers to shark cartilage as having the possibility of being ". . . the most promising weapon against tumors developed yet, and may be the "outside factor" that increases cancer cure rates form 50 percent to 80–90 percent."[7] In other words, shark cartilage targets tumors from without; meaning that it cuts off tumor blood flow, hence, the tumor shrinks rather than flourishes. It does this without destroying healthy tissue. Shark cartilage has the ability to be a much more discriminating therapy in that unlike radiation and chemotherapy, it leaves healthy tissue alone.

How does such a seemingly innocuous material like cartilage accomplish a feat that has eluded even the most brilliant modern scientist?

Tumor Angiogenesis and Shark Cartilage

A tumor is comprised of a mass of newly developed tissue whose growth has been triggered by unknown factors. Tumors can be caused by exposing normal, healthy tissue to carcinogens which can come in the form of chemicals, radiation, viruses or free radicals. Exposure alone is not always sufficient to cause the development of cancer. Cancer results only when precancerous cells are allowed to proliferate to the point where they form a system of vessels designed to sustain their continued growth. All precancerous cells do not become cancer. A strong immune system frequently checks their growth and the development of a potential tumor is prevented.

If a benign tumor forms, it is not considered a threat, although, if large enough, it can interfere with normal organ function. A cancerous or malignant tumor not only grows unchecked but can transmit cancerous cells to other body tissue via the blood or lymph—a process called metastasis. When this happen, tumor growth can occur in any part of the body these cancerous cells become lodged in.

For a tumor to survive, it must be sustained by nutrients that reach it through a network of blood vessels. Dr. Judah Folkman, M.D. of the Harvard Medical School, observed and experimented with tumor growth and concluded that:

1. Tumors cannot grow unless they have access to a network of blood vessels which provided cell nutrients and the removal of waste products from the tissue.

2. A viable cancer therapy may exist if the creation of this network of blood vessels to tumor masses could be inhibited.[8]

Dr. Folkman proposed that a tumor could be prevented from growing past the size of a pencil point if its network of blood vessels was inhibited.[9]

Dr. Folkman's findings led to the use of a term called angiogenesis, which technically refers to the creation of placental blood vessels during the course of pregnancy. The developing fetus or growing child experiences angiogenesis during normal growth, however, as adults, the process only occurs during the healing of wounds or broken bones, during the course of ovulation and pregnancy, in some heart conditions, or if a tumor or other abnormality develops. The theory Folkman held was that if angiogenesis could be stopped, the tumor would die.

The Anti-angiogenesis Activity of Cartilage

It seemed only logical to look to cartilage as a source of angiogenesis inhibition because this gristly material is without vascularization. In other words, it has no system of blood vessels, therefore, it must possess certain substances which prevent the formation of such vessels. Early research at MIT turned to the use of calf cartilage in experiments with tumors which proved to be quite encouraging and enlightening. When small pieces of cartilage were implanted into the embryos of chicks, blood vessels proliferated through all tissue except the cartilage.

Dr. Robert Langer of MIT and Dr. John Prudden, M.D. came to the conclusion that a certain factor in cartilage stopped the growth of new blood vessels in tumors.[10] Prudden conducted a number of tests over an eleven year period. At the end of the testing time he was able to report that using cartilage had achieved a "major inhibitory effect upon a wide spectrum of cancers."[11] What this meant was that cartilage therapy had evoked a complete response, which was defined as *no clinical evidence could exist that an active tumor was present for a minimum of twelve weeks.*

Dr. Brian G.M. Durie of the department of internal medicine at the University of Arizona Health Sciences in Tucson added to Prudden's research. He discovered that when bovine cartilage came in contact with tumor cells in vitro, the cells died. Durie obtained the same results using colon, ovarian, pancreatic and testicular cancer specimens.[12]

Because the amount of calf cartilage extract which could be obtained was relatively small, researchers looked to the shark. The entire exoskeleton of sharks is comprised of cartilage and sharks seem unusually protected from the development of malignancies. In addition, unlike bovine cartilage, shark cartilage is not surrounded by adipose tissue (fat). This meant that obtaining and purifying cartilage extract from the shark required a simpler process. For example: it takes 500 mg of bovine cartilage to make one ml of extract as compared to 0.5 mg of shark cartilage to produce the same amount.[13]

These facts prompted further research at MIT and the Harvard University Medical School. Clinical tests revealed that protein extracts derived from shark cartilage possess the ability to prevent blood vessel growth to tumors. In the early eighties, Dr. Langer and Dr. Anna Lee were able to isolate the mechanism involved in shark cartilage which kept tumors from thriving.[14] Moreover, they discovered that shark cartilage extract possessed the best ability to retard tumor development. More recently, researchers at California State University in Fresno have isolated four substances from shark cartilage which they believe contribute to cancer inhibition.[15] When all was said and done, shark cartilage had proven its ability to shrink tumors.

Shark Cartilage and Existing Tumors

Consider the following quote:
"Tumor blood cells are constantly breaking down and being replaced by new vessels. When the existing vessels break down in the presence of anti-angiogenesis factors, they are not replaced by new vessels and the section fed by the vessels dies (necrosis). You can see this when such a tumor is cut open. Instead of a pinkish tissue, the tissue is gray. Then it decays away and leaves an air-space. I refer to the appearance of air spaces . . . especially in large breast tumors. . .as 'the Swiss cheese effect.'"[16]

Apparently, shark cartilage extract had shown impressive results especially in breast, liver, brain and esophageal tumors with major changes observed withing four to six weeks.[17] It is nothing less than extraordinary to learn that the success rate of shark cartilage with solid tumors has been higher than 80 percent.[18]

If a tumor cannot metastasize or spread its malignant cells to other parts of the body, it can be contained. A study published in the January 3, 1991 edition of *The New England Journal of Medicine* supported the notion that without vascularization (blood vessels), metastasis is significantly inhibited. These findings emphasized what had already been discovered, which was that tumors grow and spread only if they are fed by blood vessels; and that shark cartilage inhibits the formation of blood vessels (angiogenesis).

NOTE: THE ANTI-ANGIOGENESIS ACTION OF SHARK CARTILAGE POSES NO THREAT TO WELL ESTABLISHED AND NORMAL BLOOD CAPILLARY NETWORKS IN ADULTS. ABNORMAL, NEW BLOOD VESSEL NETWORKS DEVELOP IN SPECIFIC DISEASES LIKE CERTAIN CANCERS AND CAN BE INHIBITED BY THE ACTION OF SHARK CARTILAGE IN A PERFECTLY SAFE AND NON-TOXIC MANNER.

THE CASE FOR SHARK CARTILAGE AS A CANCER THERAPY

Research at Jules Bordet Institute in Brussels

In 1988, Dr. Ghanem Atassi of the Jules Bordet Institute in Brussels conducted a dramatic experiment in which he gave 40 mice melanoma (skin cancer) grafts. Half of the mice were left medication free and the other half were given daily doses of shark cartilage. After 21 days, the tumors in the untreated mice had doubled. By contrast, the mice on shark cartilage extracts experienced a decrease in tumor size.[19] Interestingly, it was also discovered that the tumor growth in the untreated mice was not evidenced for two weeks. The research team hypothesized that it took two weeks for a new vascular system (blood vessels) to form around and within the tumor. They also believed that the tumor itself had somehow initiated the growth of this blood vessel network. Apparently, something in the composition of shark cartilage inhibited this compound released by the tumor, thereby preventing the creating of new vessels. Without these vessels, the tumor could not grow.

Mexican Studies

In his book *Sharks Don't Get Cancer*, Dr. Lane discusses clinical trial results using shark cartilage in specific cases of disease. These studies were conducted in the early nineties at the Ernesto Contreras Hospital in Mexico with the collaboration of Doctors Ernesto and Francesco Contreras, both medical physicians. Eight patients with terminal cancer or serious tumors were tested with shark cartilage alone. The following results were obtained.[20]

1) In seven out of eight patients a reduction in tumor size of 30 to 100 percent occurred.
2) A woman with stage III cervical cancer that was considered inoperable, experienced an eighty percent reduction of the tumor and almost

total eradication of pain after 7 weeks of treatment. Following 11 weeks of shark cartilage therapy, the tumor was 100 percent reduced, with no pain and only scar tissue remaining.

3) After undergoing maximum radiation treatments, a women with a vaginal hemangioma experienced a 60 percent reduction in a tumor that was the size of a grapefruit after seven weeks of treatment with shark cartilage. After eleven weeks of therapy, the tumor had shrunk further.

4) A thirty-two year old female suffering from very advanced cervical cancer with a blockage of the kidney took shark cartilage as a last resort. Her death was considered imminent. After seven weeks, the tumor had shrunk by 40 percent, and her pain was almost gone. By eleven weeks, the tumor had reduced by 60 percent.

5) A sixty-two year old female with advanced peritoneal carcinoma given little chance of survival took shark cartilage for seven weeks, after which the tumor shrunk 20 percent. At eleven weeks, she was tumor free—her case was considered a miracle cure by other physicians.

6) In Panama, a patient with an advanced liver tumor experienced a complete remission after eight weeks of shark cartilage treatment.

Additional studies consistently confirmed similar results in other patients suffering from advanced breast tumors and uterine fibroids. These findings were impressive, to say the least. It was the Cuban clinical studies which eventually drew significant media attention and was featured in 1993 on 60 Minutes, aired by CBS.

The Cuban Clinical Trials

In 1993, eighteen patients were evaluated after similar therapies combining oral and rectal administration of shark cartilage. Again, it must be remembered that each of these patients were considered gravely ill at the outset, and in some cases, were suffering from malnutrition as well. Almost 40 percent of these subjects experienced a significant improvement. Dr. Lane points out that even in the cases where a cure did not occur, the use of shark cartilage dramatically improved the quality of life.[21]

The following results were obtained with shark cartilage therapy:[22]

1) An eighty-two year old man suffering from prostate cancer that had already metastasized became pain free after two weeks on shark cartilage. At sixteen weeks, ultrasound showed a 59 percent reduction in the tumor.
2) A sixty-three year old woman with breast cancer metastasized to the chest wall became symptom free after six weeks of shark cartilage therapy.
3) A twenty-two year old man with a brain tumor, most of which had been surgically removed, experienced no re-growth on shark cartilage.
4) In Panama, a patient with an advanced liver tumor experienced what doctors refer to as a complete remission after eight weeks of shark cartilage treatment.

Shark Cartilage Shakes Up 60 Minutes

In a CBS broadcast of 60 Minutes, Mike Wallace explored the claims of shark cartilage in his usual skeptical way. He interviewed patient who were beginning a clinical study of shark cartilages as a viable cancer treatment in Cuba before and after treatment in January of 1993. All clinical results were scrutinized by the 60 Minutes staff, and in February of 1993 the program concluded that *shark cartilage therapy was a promising treatment.* [23]

NOTE: It is important to realize that shark cartilage can augment conventional cancer treatments as well as other nutritional protocols. In other words, using shark cartilage in combination with vitamin C, selenium, pycnogenol, herbs such as Taheebo, and various amino acids is recommended.

What Kinds of Cancer Respond Best to Shark Cartilage?

Clearly, extracts of shark cartilage show a great deal of potential in treating cancers which are characterized by solid tumors. Solid tumor masses require the presence of an efficient system of blood vessels to survive and are typically found in breast, cervical, pancreatic, prostate or ovarian cancer. Cancers which do not depend on blood vessel networks to survive such as inflammatory breast cancer, Hodgkin's disease or leukemia are less likely to respond to shark cartilage therapy.

AIDS and Kaposi's Sarcoma

Kaposi's sarcoma was a relatively unheard of form of cancer until AIDS became a common household word. It is a considered a rare form of cancer that is characterized by tumor cell invasion of the lining of small blood vessels. In time, if the tumors are allowed to grow, these vessels become obstructed and tissued edema and destruction occurs.

Prior to the AIDS epidemic, Kaposi's sarcoma rarely targeted young people and received little media attention. Even before AIDS arrived on the scene, doctors recognized that the disease was "opportunistic." In other words, it was the type of cancer that occurs when the immune system is greatly compromised or weakened.

Today, Kaposi's sarcoma afflicts 25 percent of all patients diagnosed with AIDS. (Subsequent autopsies of AIDS victims revealed that the tumors are present in 90 percent of those who die from AIDS.)[24]

Like so many other forms of cancer, Kaposi's sarcoma does not respond to traditional cancer therapy. Research turned to the development of drugs designed to inhibit the angiogenesis necessary for Kaposi's sarcoma to develop. Dr. I William Lane strongly believes that the anti-angiogenic action of shark cartilage could greatly benefit anyone suffering from Kaposi's sarcoma. These cancerous lesions are comprised of endothelial cells, which are the very cells shark cartilage inhibits. In addition, these tumors are characterized by heavy vessel formation, which is exactly what shark cartilage stops.

Interestingly, using shark cartilage for AIDS related diseases like Kaposi's sarcoma may actually potentiate and augment conventional radiation therapy. Dr. Lane writes about a young man suffering from AIDS and Kaposi's sarcoma and shark cartilage therapy:

Michael Callanan, author of Surviving AIDS *was diagnosed as having AIDS in the early 1980s. Eventually, KS lesions covered more that two-thirds of his lungs. The chemotherapy prescribed to fight his KS had such "horrible" side effects that Michael called a halt to them. Two months later, he learned of an opening in a clinical trail being conducted by Eric Flerishman, M.D., of Los Angeles. Michael entered the program and began taking shark cartilage. He also elected to undergo radiation therapy despite warnings that "it was not a very good idea" (radiation might further compromise his immune* system) and that he should "not expect anything." Neither the radiologist nor the technician knew that he was taking shark cartilage.

Michael's right lung was treated in sessions using 1,000 rads, a relatively low dose. When the course of treatment was complete, that lung was completely clear, but Michael's left lung had gotten worse. The left lung was also treated with radiation for ten days, after which both lungs were completely clear of KS lesions.

Health care professional involved with Michael believe that the shark cartilage acted as a radiation potentiator. Further evidence of cartilage's ability to augment the effect of radiation came when Michael had treatment for lesions on his legs.. The plan had been for him to receive a normal dose of 2,000 rads. At 1,200 rads, a dose normally free from side effects, he began to exhibit radiation burns. Michael, therefore, urges those taking shark cartilage to inform their radiologists. He also recommends that shark-cartilage users begin with low doses of radiation.[25]

How Much Cartilage is Needed to Treat Cancer?

Dr. Lane findings were based on using 60 grams of whole shark cartilage per day based on a body weight of under 140 pounds. In advanced cases, he has used up to 120 grams daily.[26] Between 60 and 80 grams per day is typically prescribed.

Prevention of Recurring Cancer

According to the research of Dr. Lane and other physicians, it appears that 7 to 8 grams of shark cartilage taken daily may prevent the recurrence of tumors. Using shark cartilage as a preventative therapeutic holds great promise and has remained relatively unexplored. It has become obvious, however, that in order to control certain tumorous conditions and angiogenic diseases, shark cartilage must be taken for an indefinite period of time.

How Shark Cartilage Boosts the Immune System

In the process of testing shark cartilage as an effective treatment for cancer and other tumors, various unexpected and beneficial side effects emerged. Oriental medical practitioners have used shark cartilage to increase stamina and boost resistance to disease. Recent research has discovered that certain biochemicals called mucopolysaccharides and anti-angiogenesis compounds actually work to prevent diseases.[27] These mucopolysaccharides stimulate the immune system. In addition, the protein components of shark cartilage complement these carbohydrates to fight off disease, while the phosphorus and calcium content serve as metabolic nutrients. The complementary and synergistic action of all of the chemical constituents of shark cartilage would prompt the assumption that it is best to take shark cartilage in its entirety, rather than attempting to separate its therapeutic components.

Shark Cartilage and Arthritis

An added bonus in evaluating the ability of shark cartilage to reduce tumors was discovering that another of its primary effects is in reducing pain. The type of pain that results from the presence of a tumor or joint inflammation seems particularly vulnerable to shark cartilage. Interestingly, angiogenesis not only occurs to sustain tumors, but also in diabetic retinopathy, certain types of glaucoma and rheumatoid arthritis.

Rheumatoid and osteoarthritis afflict more than 30 million Americans. Rheumatoid arthritis is considered an autoimmune disease in which the body's defense systems actually attacks itself. The result is the continual inflammation of joints. It is estimated that between 1 and 3 percent of the population will suffer from arthritis at one time or another.

Arthritis can be an extremely debilitating disease which causes an inordinate amount of suffering worldwide. The disease process creates joint defects, immobility, muscle wasting, and bone and cartilage destruction. Like cancer, the outlook for curing rheumatoid arthritis has been rather dim. Treatment usually involves targeting symptoms with various pain killers or non-steroidal anti-inflammatory drugs like ibuprofen and other NSAIDs, which come with significant side effects.

While the cause of arthritis eludes medical science, the abnormal creation of tiny capillaries has been observed as the disease unfolds. This blood vessel network can eventually destroy the cartilage that cushions the joints and significantly contribute to the pain and joint destruction typical of arthritis. Dr. Lane compares this phenomenon with water that gets into the cracks of concrete, freezes and expands, thereby eventually breaking up the cement. These unwanted blood vessels cause a similar effect within cartilage tissue. The evolution of arthritic joint blood vessels is another example of angiogenesis. It only stands to reason that if shark cartilage possess anti-angiogenic properties, it must be valuable for arthritic conditions.

Arthritic Angiogenesis and Shark Cartilage

Various data derived from animal studies and clinical studies applied to humans has shown the efficacy of shark cartilage in treating arthritis.[28] Dr. Jose A. Orcasita, M.D., tested the effectiveness of shark cartilage extract on several arthritis sufferers, who experienced significant improvement. Subsequent studies at the University of Miami School of Medicine found that arthritic pain could be substantially decreased by using shark cartilage extract. Dr. Orcasita stressed the fact that patients who took shark cartilage for arthritis experienced no side effects or toxicity of any kind. Dr. Lane's findings support the use of shark cartilage for arthritis. Shark cartilage targets arthritis in two ways:

1. It works as a natural anti-inflammatory helping to ease joint inflammation.
2. As arthritis evolves, an abnormal network of blood vessels can develop in inflamed regions. These vessels substantially contributes to the extreme pain and stiffness associated with arthritis. As previously discusses, shark cartilage significantly inhibits the creation of blood vessels.

A New Kind of Anti-Inflammatory Agent

While shark cartilage does not have the ability to restore damaged cartilage or bone, it can help to control inflammation and is particularly good for pain control.

Shark cartilage appears to block the angiogenic process, and thereby significantly reduces joint inflammation and pain. These effects are achieved in part because of the large and effective amounts of mucopolysaccharides contained in shark cartilage. In almost all cases, the immobility and pain of arthritis are a result of inflammation. The inflammation-fighting mucopolysaccharides work with the angiogenesis-inhibiting proteins to produce a response that is much more significant than the response wither might produce if working alone. This synergistic effect stops inflammation, pain and further breakdown of the cartilage. Several clinical studies support these theories.[29]

Health practitioners strongly believe that shark cartilage will revolutionize the treatment of arthritis as a safe and practical therapy. Unlike NSAIDs, which comprise the standard medical treatment for joint pain, shark cartilage is safe and non-toxic to the body.

Side Effects of Drugs Used for Arthritis

NSAIDs include ibuprofen, eiflunisal, salicylate, indomethacin, eiflunisal and tolmetin. More common trade names are: Advil, Tylenol, Aleve, Motrin, Naprosyn, etc. This category of drug is one of the most widely prescribed in the United States. Obviously, pain has become a way of life for most Americans. Unfortunately, because of their accessibility and the free manner in which these drugs are prescribed, they are taken liberally and for everything from a slight headache to severe arthritic pain. Some of the side effects of NSAIDs include peptic ulcers, hemorrhage, stomach problems, ear ringing, dizziness, low blood sugar, kidney dysfunction and abnormal heart rhythms.

Ibuprofen-based products should not be taken if you have kidney trouble, or if you are pregnant or nursing. In addition, mixing ibuprofen with aspirin or alcohol can be risky. Millions of people take NSAIDs daily and thousands become sick or even die from NSAIDs-related side effects.

By contrast, shark cartilage may offer a significant therapeutic benefit for arthritis sufferers without the deleterious side effects of NSAIDs and steroid drugs. Sadly, very few victims of arthritis are aware of shark cartilage and its impressive effect on the disease.

CASE STUDIES USING SHARK CARTILAGE FOR ARTHRITIS

Dr. John Prudden's work in the early seventies supported the notion that cartilage treatment of twenty-eight arthritic patients conditions showed impressive results with no adverse side effects. Nineteen of those treated who had suffered severe pain or dysfunction obtained "excellent" results.[30]

In 1988, Dr. Serge Orloff, a prominent, European arthritis specialist, obtained similar results using shark cartilage. Subsequent Eastern European studies found that in some patients:

> *arthritic pain could be decreased by 50 percent or more
> *a marked improvement in the quality of life was observed
> *increased function and activity resulted
> *bedridden patients became ambulatory[31]

In Panama, Dr. Harry Xatrush, M.D. added to the clinical data by using shark cartilage for a painful back and hip condition. After eighteen days of therapy, a marked improvement occurred with the elimination of morning stiffness and muscle cramping.[32] Another patient who had taken analgesics, NSAIDs, immunosuppressants, steroids and other less conventional medicines took shark cartilage for 21 days. Surprisingly, he was able to straighten his spine and his pain was totally gone. He states:

My spine has straightened out; I am able to move my arms and legs without pain; my walk has improved; I am more agile. I feel like working; I'm not tired and my constipation and gastritis have improved.[33]

Dr. Alpizar of Costa Rica used oral administrations of shark cartilage for 10 patients who were bedridden with severe cases of osteoarthritis. Within three weeks, eight out of ten were mobile.[34] In addition, a survey of patients who used shark cartilage for arthritis demonstrated that 140 out of 158 persons reported, excellent, fair or good results.[35]

In order to dismiss the notion that these test results may have been psychosomatic or based on the placebo effect, subsequent testing with dogs was conducted in 1991. All of the dogs suffered from extreme osteoarthritis confirmed in all of their cases as resulting from earlier accidents or normal aging. Measurements were based on six criteria, three functional like the ability to move or to jump over and obstacle, and three nonfunctional, like swelling and joint pain. The dogs were given the shark cartilage daily in their food for three weeks. In the functional (active) criteria, all showed at least a 50 percent improvement in three weeks, while with the nonfunctional criteria, swelling or inflammation decreased by 70 percent. There were no side effects and in all cases the owners described their dogs as much more active and even happier.[36]

The bottom line is that shark cartilage should be considered a viable alternative to the use of steroids and NSAIDs for arthritis inflammation and pain. It has proven to be successful in reducing pain in approximately 70 percent of osteoarthritis cases and 60 percent in cases of rheumatoid arthritis. These statistics are nothing less than extraordinary.

Psoriasis

Psoriasis is another baffling physiologic condition which involves the abnormal proliferation of new blood vessels in the skin. It afflicts millions of people and is unusually difficult to control and treat. Psoriasis occurs when skin cell production gets out of control, much in the same way that tumor cells proliferate. This abnormal production of skin cells causes the formation of thick skin patches, sometimes referred to as plaques.

Conventional medical treatments for psoriasis include the use of corticosteroids, coal tar, ultraviolet light and in severe cases, a drug called methotrexate, which poses considerable health risks to the liver. None of these treatments is considered very effective, and the disease is still classified as incurable.

How often does the option of shark cartilage therapy arise when discussing psoriasis? The assumption that the skin thickening and shedding typical of psoriasis may depend on the abnormal formation of capillaries directs the disease to shark cartilage therapy. The anti-angiogenic action of shark cartilage has proved to be an effective treatment for the disease Shark cartilage has the ability to help control psoriasis and contributes to the fading of psoriasis patches.

Dr. Prudden in his work with shark cartilage obtained a remarkable measure of success with thirty-nine patients suffering from psoriasis.[37] Using injections of Catrix-S, a special cartilage product, he was able to affect significant improvement in the majority of cases. Out of 30 patients in his test group, 19 experienced total remission with psoriasis patches and lesion disappearing for six weeks to one year.[38] Of the sixteen who did not experience a complete remission, fifteen had what they could consider good results.[39] Eventually, eleven of these patients did achieve a remission after additional injections.

Dr. Julian Whitaker, M.D. is a strong advocate of shark cartilage for severe cases of psoriasis. He states:

Jane was 65 and had as bad a case of psoriasis as I have seen. Her legs were solid with fiery red patches, which were also on her chest, back and arms. She had seen a university-based dermatologist without success; her visit to me was a last resort. I started her on a shark cartilage supplement, and her improvement was immediate and miraculous, Her arms in turn cleared completely, and the legs cleared to just a few bald patches.[40]

Concerning the treatment of psoriasis, Dr. Lane writes:

. . .the effective dosage level for psoriasis is 15-20 grams daily depending on body weight, Be aware that with this treatment, the itching and scales will be the first symptoms to disappear. Without the scales, the redness of the skin will appear to intensify since the large bed of capillary vessels will be more apparent. This capillary bed will also slowly disappear over a period of sixty to ninety days.

Enteritis and other Intestinal Disorders

Dr. Prudden also used cartilage to successfully treat enteritis, which is an inflammation of the bowel lining. Dr. Lane points out that, ". . .in a 1991 study in southern California at the Comprehensive Medical Clinic, two patients with Candida enteritis responded quickly to shark cartilage administered orally at the rate of 9 grams per day."[42]

Interestingly, shark cartilage has been effective in treating a variety of conditions characterized by intestinal inflammation. Consider the following quote:

The administration of shark cartilage has yielded very good response with all sorts of intestinal inflammation. A doctor on the West Coast once told me that he advised many of his patients with intestinal inflammation to use shark cartilage as a food supplement.[43]

As with other conditions, taking shark cartilage throughout the day and before meals seems to be the most effective method.

Poison Oak and Poison Ivy

During the coarse of Dr. Prudden's work with psoriasis patients, he discovered that cases of poison oak and ivy also responded well to shark cartilage therapy. One case in particular was extremely severe and was characterized by unusually bad itching, edema and peeling skin. Traditional treatments and prescription ointments had failed to bring any relief. Dr. Prudden treated the affected skin with Catrix (shark cartilage) ointment and relief was almost immediate. Within five minutes, the itching had ceased, and within two weeks the skin was normal.[44] Interestingly, Dr. Prudden experimented with using the cream as a protectant against poison ivy before exposure to the plant. Applying the cream served to protect the skin. No allergic reaction developed.[45]

In addition to psoriasis, poison ivy and oak, success with cartilage therapy was also obtained in cases of acne, mandibular alveolitis (dry socket), a condition which can occur after a tooth extraction, hemorrhoids and chronic anal itching.[46]

Diabetic Retinopathy, Neovascular Glaucoma, and Macular Degeneration: Three Major Causes of Blindness

Diabetic retinopathy occurs when tiny blood vessels and capillaries rupture within the retina leaving behind a deposit. The subsequent initiation of an abnormal network of new blood vessels occurs and causes a slow and progressive loss of vision. Diabetic retinopathy is one of the most common causes of blindness and is a risk for most insulin dependent diabetics. Scientists who have observed the ability of shark cartilage to stop the creation of blood vessels believe that it can prevent the course of retinopathy and may also affect neoevascular glaucoma in the same way. This type of glaucoma occurs when pressure in the eyeball is increased due to the abnormal presence of blood vessel networks.

For adults over sixty-five, macular degeneration is a primary cause of permanent blindness. It occurs when a region near the retina deteriorates. In some cases, this deterioration is preceded by a proliferation of blood vessels that leak fluid into the retina causing scar tissue and eventual loss of vision. If optical examinations detect these leaky vessels early enough, they can be removed or cauterized, a process which is very difficult and can easily damage healthy retinal tissue. The procedure is costly and poses a significant risk.

Researchers believe that using shark cartilage could prevent macular degeneration from occurring in the first place. As a preventative agent, shark cartilage could be administered to anyone who had a predisposition for these three sight robbing diseases.

Other Diseases that May Respond to Shark Cartilage

Because shark cartilage is rich in mucopolysaccharides, diseases which are associated with changes in this large molecule may also benefit from shark cartilage therapy. Disease which may respond favorably to shark cartilage therapy include: acne, eczema, anal itching, atherosclerosis, colitis, gastritis, asthma, poison oak, poison ivy, emphysema, and hemorrhoids.

The Quality of Shark Cartilage Supplements

During an interview with Richard Passwater, Dr. Lane stated:
In late 1992, two separate proteins, both with major angiogenic properties have been identified, one by Dr. Robert Langer and a second by Japanese researchers.[47] *It is postulated that as many as five separate active anti-angiogenic proteins are in shark cartilage. With the whole shark cartilage properly prepared, all work synergistically. Proteins are easily denatured (inactivated by heat, acids, alcohols, acetones and many other chemicals. This proper processing to prevent denaturization is most important.*[48]

Some have wondered why the angiogenesis protein components of shark cartilage have not been extracted and used in an isolated form. Evidently, this very task is what may be what is holding up the classification of shark cartilage as a viable medicine. It is vital to understand, however, that like so many other natural substances like bee pollen, herbs, etc., the entire chemical makeup of shark cartilage creates a synergistic unit. The proteins, carbohydrates and minerals found in shark cartilage complement and augment each other. Unlike synthetic pharmaceutical preparations which have been chemically synthesized and altered, shark cartilage is best taken as nature created it.

Look for shark cartilage extract that has been properly processed and comes from a proven and reliable source. It should be 100 percent pure whole shark cartilage with no fillers or binders and should offer a concentration that can be used in practical therapeutic dosages.

NOTE: As more publicity surfaces regarding shark cartilage as a viable treatment for cancer, demand will inevitably increase and costs will mushroom. Watch for reliable products from credible sources.

Forms of Shark Cartilage

Shark cartilage is available in desiccated, dried, loose powder forms and should be mixed with fruit juice or water. It can also be taken in gel caps or as a liquid supplement. Shark oils or shark cartilage is also available in topical ointment or cream forms due to its healing and protective properties. As mentioned, potency is an issue and shark cartilage forms should be purchased which can provide practical therapeutic dosages for the best price.

Effective Ways of Consuming Shark Cartilage

Typically, shark cartilage is taken orally within a juice medium throughout the day before meals. After the tumor has decreased or is no longer present, using 10 to 15 grams of shark cartilage daily is recommended for prevention for an unspecified length of time. Enemas or injections of shark cartilage should be used only under the supervision of a physician. Taking shark cartilage as a preventative against macular degeneration or other diseases which rely on the process of angiogenesis may also be warranted in some cases where genetic predisposition exists.

Shark Cartilage and Safety

Concerning the safety of shark cartilage, Dr. Lane has stated:

Shark cartilage. . .like all active material. . .must be used properly. Since it inhibits new vascularization, those having suffered a recent coronary occlu-

sion (heart attack) pregnant women and those wanting to conceive, and people recovering from recent surgery should all refrain from use for a logical time period. We have experienced some stomach upsets, primarily with those on a macrobiotic or vegetarian diet who also respond more slowly. We see some very limited allergic responses, but in general, most people can use shark cartilage with no problems at all."[49] The Chinese have consumed shark fin soup for generations. Taking shark cartilage for an extended period may may affect the rate in which a wound or incision heals. There is also a possibility that conception is impaired when shark cartilage is used for prolonged periods. The side effects of prolonged inhibition of capillary growth in healthy adults are unknown...it appears that delayed wound healing and contraception may be among the few detectable side effects of therapy lasting eight weeks or more.[50]

NOTE: PREGNANT WOMEN, THOSE ATTEMPTING TO CONCEIVE, ANYONE WHO HAS RECENTLY HAD SURGERY (ESPECIALLY HEART SURGERY), OR HAS EXPERIENCED A HEART ATTACK, OR ANYONE RECOVERING FROM AN INJURY SHOULD NOT TAKE SHARK CARTILAGE. BECAUSE CHILDREN ARE STILL IN PHYSIOLOGICAL DEVELOPMENT, THEY SHOULD NOT TAKE SHARK CARTILAGE.

Shark Cartilage and Environmental Concerns

When asked if sharks might become an endangered species as a result of shark cartilage therapy, it was pointed out that approximately 10 million sharks are harvested each year for shark-fin soup usage alone. If the exoskeletons of these sharks were kept rather than discarded, enough shark cartilage would exist to treat 625,000 cancer patients yearly without killing one additional shark.[51]

Shark Cartilage Has Earned Its Patent

Apparently, obtaining a patent is no easy task. Convincing evidence must be amassed and presented in order for a patent to be issued for any health-food supplement. As a result, patenting natural supplements is relatively rare; not because the supplements are not effective but because clinical testing is often out of reach or non-existent. Shark cartilage is one of the few substances that is patented due to mainly two reasons: that CAM assay proves the ability of shark cartilage to inhibit angiogenesis; and that Xenograft studies support the angiogenic activity of shark cartilage.

Dr. I. William Lane received a patent for shark cartilage on Dec. 24, 1991. Part of that patent referring to the action of shark cartilage reads as follows:

This invention relates generally to a method of and a dosage unit for inhibiting angiogenesis or vascularization in an animal having an intestinal wall utilizing an effective amount of shark cartilage, particularly finely divided shark cartilage, for passing though the intestinal wall as a suspension for inhibiting interalia, tumor growth and metastasis, in particular Kaposi sarcoma, arthritis, in particular rheumatoid arthritis, diabetic retinopathy and neovascular glaucoma, psoriasis, and inflammatory diseases with vascular component.[52]

Shark Cartilage and Preventative Therapy

Unfortunately, our medical system is based on the idea of "putting out fires rather than preventing them." In other words, the notion of prevention is rarely addressed. Once disease mechanisms have taken hold, medical practitioners attempt to stay their course by using radical and harmful therapies or by prescribing potent pain killing drugs to mask their symptoms.

Shark cartilage has the potential to prevent the development of diseases requiring angiogenesis. This is profoundly important and could change significantly change the course of diseases like cancer. Because it is a completely non-toxic and safe food supplement, its prophylactic usage should be evaluated and applied. It could save countless lives.

MEDICINAL APPLICATIONS OF SHARK CARTILAGE

- *acne*
- *asthma*
- *cancer (breast, cervix, Kaposi's*
- *arthritis*
- *atherosclerosis*

sarcoma, prostate, pancreatic, ovarian
and testicular in particular)
- *colitis*
- *eczema*
- *glaucoma (neovascular)*
- *diabetic retinopathy*
- *high blood pressure*
- *Kaposi's sarcoma*
- *poison ivy and poison oak*
- *pruritus ani (intense anal itching)*
- *wound healing*

- *cataracts*
- *emphysema*
- *gastritis*
- *enteritis*
- *hemorrhoids*
- *joint inflammation*
- *mandibular alveolitis*
- *psoriasis*
- *skin disorders*

The Untapped Medicinal Potential of Shark Cartilage

Currently, worldwide research continues on this remarkable substance. Unfortunately, established medical practitioners and research scientists have been slow to admit that the impressive tract record shark cartilage has amassed should be aggressively published and its applications pursued. It remains classified as a food supplement and not an accepted medicine. On April 29, 1992, the National Cancer Institute announced that it would not fund shark cartilage testing because the studies were not "impressive" enough (one has to wonder what their definition of "impressive" is). Clearly, the clinical studies discussed in this booklet have been enormously impressive. As mentioned earlier, we are not winning our war with cancer in spite of billions of expended dollars. Each and every year, millions of people become cancer statistics and are continually failed by traditional treatments. Shark cartilage has shown its medicinal muscle. At the very least, it should be tried, especially in cases where conventional therapies have failed. It is a potentially curative, non-toxic substance and should be included as an augmentive therapy to any medical treatment protocol.

Aside from its value for cancer, arthritis and psoriasis, shark cartilage holds a medicinal promise for speedier wound healing, possible advances in cataract surgery, and new therapies for high blood pressure and heart failure. Richard P. Huemer, M.D. writes:

Scientists are interested in isolating and synthesizing the anti-angiogenesis factors in shark cartilage, with an eye toward drug development; but, some people wonder why we have to wait for all that. Purified shark cartilage is available now, it appears to work, and it's non-toxic. There appears to be no harm in using it alongside more conventional treatments to alleviate the suffering of chronic illness.[53]

Dr. Lane adds his observations:

. . .although the scientific detectives know that they were on to something, their training had them conditioned to look for a pure chemical that could be isolated, synthesized and patented.

Dr. Lane has applied for and recently received full FDA permission to continue with the second phase of clinical trials on shark cartilage in cases of non-responsive prostate cancer and Kaposi's sarcoma. Lane will be conducting these tests at a leading center. He is hopeful that positive test data will lead to FDA approval of shark cartilage as an accepted cancer treatment.

Despite media coverage and sporadic publicity, shark cartilage remains relatively unknown to the general public. Sadly, its life-saving properties remain a secret for thousands of individuals who might profoundly benefit from its therapeutic actions. Unquestionably, shark cartilage will eventually emerge as an exciting and legitimate cancer treatment. When it does, one can be certain that while its availability may increase, it will become a prescription drug and its cost will dramatically rise.

While the concept of anti-angiogenesis has been praised by the scientific community, further research and development of shark cartilage has been slow. The evidence is conclusive, impressive and even startling. Shark cartilage is out there, however, its life-saving potential remains untapped. Millions of people suffering from cancer and other debilitating diseases continue to subject themselves to radical conventional treatments, totally unaware of the existence of shark cartilage therapy. At the very least, shark cartilage should augment standard therapies for cancer, arthritis, psoriasis and so on. Education is the key and knowledge creates options. Clearly, shark cartilage is a remarkable breakthrough therapy.

ENDNOTES

[1] Dr. I. William Lane and Linda Comac. SHARKS DON'T GET CANCER. (Avery Publishing, Garden City, New York: 1993), 76.
[2] Ibid., 37.
[3] Ibid., 43.
[4] Richard A. Passwater, Ph.D. CANCER PREVENTION AND NUTRITIONAL THERAPIES. (Keats Publishing, New Canaan, Connecticut: 1978), 97.
[5] Arnold Fox, M.D. and Nadine Taylor, M.S., R.D. "The Wonders of Shark Cartilage." LET'S LIVE. (March, 1994), 14.
[6] Ibid.
[7] Passwater, 111.
[8] Lane, 40. See also "Tumor angiogenesis." THE NEW ENGLAND JOURNAL OF MEDICINE, (1971) 285:1182-86.
[9] Judah Folkman. "Tumor angiogenesis: Therapeutic implications." NEW ENGLAND JOURNAL OF MEDICINE. (1971) 285:1182-6.
[10] Robert Langer et al., "Isolation of a cartilage factor that inhibits tumor neovascularization," SCIENCE. (1976) 193:70-72. See also Anne lee and Robert Langer. "Shark cartilage contains inhibitors of tumor angiogenesis." SCIENCE (1983) 221:1185-87, and John F. Prudden. "The treatment of human cancer with agents prepared from bovine cartilage." JOURNAL OF BIOLOGICAL RESPONSE MODIFIERS. (1985) 4:551-84.
[11] Fox, 15.
[12] Ibid.
[13] Ibid.
[14] Lee and Langer. "Shark cartilage contains inhibitors of tumor angiogenesis," 1185-87.
[15] Otis Port. "Maybe Jaws Can Put the Bite on Cancer." BUSINESS WEEK. (Nov. 21, 1994) 3400, 93.
[16] Passwater, 99.
[17] Ibid., 100.
[18] Ibid., 102.
[19] Fox, 15.
[20] Ibid., 16.
[21] Lane, 102.
[22] Fox, 16.
[23] Passwater, 104.
[24] Lane, 83.
[25] Ibid., 83-84.
[26] Passwater, 101.
[27] Richard P. Huemer. "Shark cartilage has brought relief to cancer pain." LET'S LIVE. (April, 1995) 63:4, 56.
[28] Gary Gagliardi. "Shark cartilage for achy joints." MUSCLE AND FITNESS. (Oct. 1995) 56:10, 52-57.
[29] Lane, 117.
[30] Ibid.
[31] Lane, 117-120.
[32] Ibid., 123.
[33] Ibid., 124.
[34] Fox, 16.
[35] Julian Whitaker, M.D. DR. WHITAKER'S GUIDE TO NATURAL HEALING. (Prima

Publishing, Rocklin, California: 1995), 341.
[36] "Shark Cartilage, an Interview with Dr. I. William Lane." HEALTHY TIMES. (Nov.-Dec., 1992), 26.
[37] Lane, 127.
[38] Fox, 18.
[39] Lane, 128.
[40] Whitaker, 334.
[41] Lane, 131.
[42] Ibid.
[43] Ibid.
[44] Ibid., 129.
[45] Ibid., 130.
[46] Ibid.
[47] Marsha A. Moses, Judith Sudhalter and Robert Langer. "Identification of an inhibitor of neovascularization from cartilage." SCIENCE. (1990) 248:1408-10. See also H. Oihawa et. Al., "A novel angiogenic inhibitor derived from Japanese shark cartilage." CANCER LETTERS. (1990) 51:181-86.
[48] Passwater, 98.
[49] Ibid., 102.
[50] Lane, 134.
[51] Passwater, 102-03.
[52] Lane, 79.
[53] Huemer, 56.